TAKE CARE OF YOURSELF

A Real-World Guide to Reclaiming Your Peace, Power, and Purpose

By

Mason Reed

Published by Eagle Eye Press Cover design by Abdul Graphics
Printed in the United States of America

First Edition
ISBN: 979-8-9928316-3-4
For inquiries: masonreedbooks@gmail.com

Dedication

To the overthinkers, over-givers, and overcomers—this is for you. You've held it together long enough.

Now it's time to take care of you.

Table of Contents

Introduction

If you're reading this, I want you to know something right away:

You're not crazy. You're just tired.

You're not broken. You've just been carrying too much for too long.

And you're not weak—you've just forgotten how strong it is to stop and say, "I matter too."

This book was written for the person who always shows up. For the one who holds everything together.

For the one who smiles through stress and says, "I'm good" when deep down, you're not.

You've probably spent most of your life taking care of everybody else. Being dependable. Being the glue. Being the strong one.

But somewhere in that process... you stopped showing up for you. You stopped listening to your body.

You stopped checking in with your mind.

You stopped nurturing your peace.

And now, you're burned out, numb, overwhelmed, and maybe even a little lost.

I know the feeling well. Because I've been there. I've lived it.

And I've learned that healing doesn't happen when you ignore yourself—it happens when you decide to come home to yourself again.

This is Your Permission Slip

This book isn't about being perfect.

It's not about having it all together or becoming some ultra-zen version of yourself.

This is about getting real. It's about learning to say:

- "I don't have to be everything for everyone."

- "I can rest and still be valuable."

- "I can say no without guilt."

- "I can feel joy again—on my terms."

- "I deserve to take care of me."

This is your permission to let go of the weight. To stop apologizing for your needs.

To stop abandoning yourself to keep everyone else comfortable.

Because you matter.

Not when you accomplish something. Not when you fix everything.

Not when you're strong enough to handle it all. You matter now. As you are.

What You'll Find in These Pages

Each chapter in this book is designed to help you:

- Identify what's been draining you

- Break toxic thought patterns

- Reclaim your energy

- Build better boundaries

- Stop glorifying burnout

- Restore your relationship with rest, joy, and purpose

- And most importantly—remember who you are underneath the exhaustion

At the end of every chapter, you'll find Take Care Action Steps—simple, practical ways to apply what you've just read. These aren't homework assignments; they're opportunities. Moments for you to finally start prioritizing the one person you've been neglecting for too long: you.

A Note From Me to You

This isn't just a book. It's a mirror. It's a moment of truth.

It's a map back to peace.

If you feel like you've been barely making it…

If you've forgotten what it feels like to wake up without stress in your chest… If you've been performing, surviving, pretending, or burning out silently…

I want you to know that you don't have to live that way anymore. There's more for you.

More peace. More clarity. More joy.

And it all begins when you finally say, "I'm going to take care of myself now." So let's begin.

No guilt. No shame. No more putting yourself last.

Let this be the moment everything changes. You ready?

Let's go.

— Mason Reed

"You don't have to earn your worth. You already matter—right now, as you are."

Chapter 1

You Matter More Than You Know

You've been everything for everybody; reliable, strong, present. But somehow, you've lost sight of your own worth in the shuffle.

There's a quiet kind of exhaustion that creeps in—not just physical, but emotional and mental. It's what happens when you show up for everyone else but slowly stop showing up for yourself.

We live in a culture that rewards hustle and downplays rest. It applauds the grind and scoffs at gentleness. But here's what they don't tell you: you can't give your best when you're running on empty.

And more importantly—you don't have to earn your worth by how much you produce, how many people you help, or how strong you pretend to be. You matter simply because you're here.

That's where taking care of yourself begins: by remembering that your life has value—not for what you do, but for who you are.

The Truth They Don't Say Out Loud You matter.

Not when you hit that goal.

Not once you get it all figured out. Not when you finally feel "enough."

You matter now.

The moment you start to believe that, everything changes—how you set boundaries, how you rest, how you speak to yourself, how you let go of things that no longer serve you.

Because when you believe you matter, you stop running on fumes and start living from fullness. Real Talk

You might be the strong one. The dependable one.

The "I got it" one.

But even you need space to heal, breathe, and be.

This book isn't just about bubble baths and journaling (though both are great). It's about rediscovering your own permission to take care of you—without guilt, shame, or apology.

There's a version of you that nobody sees.

The version that's smiling in public but secretly screaming inside. The version that keeps showing up for work, for family, for friends—while quietly fading in the background of your own life.

You've learned to perform strength like it's a routine. You brush off compliments, downplay your needs, and make excuses for not prioritizing yourself. Not because you don't care, but because somewhere along the way, you believed your needs didn't matter as much as everyone else's.

And that belief?

It's dangerous.

It's deceptive.

It's draining.

The Lie That Got In

Society tells us—especially those who've been the "go-to" person all their lives—that self-worth is measured by output.

You're valuable if you're productive. You're lovable if you're low-maintenance.

You're strong if you're silent about your struggles.

But here's the truth: your value has nothing to do with your performance. Your value is not conditional.

It's not tied to how many people need you. It's not based on how much you accomplish. It's not rooted in perfection.

You matter simply because you exist.

And until you believe that, everything else you try to build—boundaries, healing, confidence—will feel like it's built on sand.

The Risk of Neglecting Yourself

Neglect doesn't always look like falling apart.

Sometimes, it looks like being busy. Helpful. High-functioning.

But beneath that polished surface is exhaustion that doesn't go away.

Here are signs you've been neglecting yourself:

- You feel guilty resting when things "aren't done"
- You say yes when your body and soul are begging you to say no
- You feel invisible in rooms you pour your energy into
- You're easily triggered by small things and don't know why
- You've lost touch with what actually brings you joy

This is where we pause—not to shame ourselves, but to wake up to a deeper truth: you cannot pour from a cup that's cracked.

You deserve to be whole, and your journey to wholeness begins by recognizing your worth.

Your Healing Starts With One Thought

You matter. Not "someday." Not when everything's fixed. Not after you lose the weight, earn the degree, clean the house, or make everyone else happy.

You matter now.

Taking care of yourself is not an act of rebellion. It's not a luxury. It's not selfish. It's survival. It's sustainability. It's sacred.

Because if you don't take care of yourself—who will?

Let's Get Real: Who Told You You Didn't? Ask yourself:

- When did I first learn to shrink to make others comfortable?
- Who made me feel like my feelings were "too much"?
- When did I start seeing rest as weakness?
- What am I afraid will happen if I start prioritizing myself?

Most of us were never taught how to care for ourselves—emotionally, mentally, and spiritually. We were taught to survive. To cope. To be strong.

But you weren't created to live your whole life in survival mode. You're allowed to live, not just last.

The First Step to Wholeness

The first chapter of healing begins with permission. Permission to be seen.

Permission to be tired. Permission to stop pretending.

Permission to choose yourself—especially when you're usually the last one on your own list.

You matter.

And when you believe that—really believe it—you'll stop settling for crumbs and start building a life where you are no longer overlooked, undervalued, or overused.

Take Care Action Steps

1. Daily Mirror Statement

   Every morning this week, look in the mirror and say: "I matter today. I don't need to earn rest. I don't need to prove my worth. I matter right now."

2. Reflect and Write: In your journal, answer this:

   What would my life look like if I truly believed I mattered as much as everyone else I cared for?

3. Silent Self-Check:

   Throughout your day, pause and ask yourself: "What do I need right now?"

   Then—listen to your body. And honor it, even in a small way.

4. Reclaim 30 Minutes for You:

   Block off 30 minutes this week for something that brings you peace or joy—reading, resting, walking, painting, doing nothing. Don't cancel it. Protect it like you would a meeting.

5. Affirm It Until You Believe It: Write this on a sticky note or phone wallpaper: "I matter. I choose to take care of me."

"Just because you're functioning doesn't mean you're okay. Listen to what your soul has been whispering."

Chapter 2

The Silent Burnout

You can be functioning and still be breaking down.

You can laugh, post selfies, reply to texts, show up to work—and still be burned out in ways no one sees.

That's the deception of silent burnout: it hides in plain sight. You look like you've got it all together. But inside, you're one missed call, one canceled plan, or one emotional moment away from crumbling.

This chapter is for the people who've been running on autopilot. You're not lazy. You're not unmotivated.

You're tired in a way that sleep can't fix. What Burnout Really Feels Like

Burnout isn't just about being tired. It's when tiredness becomes your identity.

It's when you start to forget what it feels like to be genuinely joyful, peaceful, excited—or even just okay.

Burnout feels like:

- Getting 8 hours of sleep and still waking up exhausted
- Dreading conversations because your emotional bandwidth is gone
- Feeling numb to the things that used to bring you joy
- Being short-tempered over things that wouldn't have bothered you before
- Crying over something small, then apologizing for "being dramatic"

- Feeling stuck, but too tired to fix anything

Silent burnout doesn't always scream. It whispers:

"Just make it through the day." "Keep your head down."

"Don't bother anyone with this."

"You're too tired to start over, just push through."

The Mental Weight You Carry

Burnout is the result of carrying too much for too long without a break or a place to release it.

It could be:

- The weight of everyone else's expectations
- The emotional load of being the strong one
- The mental checklist that never ends
- The fear that if you stop moving, it'll all fall apart

You've trained yourself to be "on" all the time.

But now? Your system is overloaded. And your soul knows it. Signs You've Been Burning Out Silently

You may not even notice it happening because you've normalized the dysfunction. Here are some signs to watch for:

- You're constantly irritated but don't know why
- You feel disconnected from your passions, goals, or even yourself
- You procrastinate everything, not from laziness but from depletion
- You feel resentment building up toward people you love
- You fantasize about running away, disappearing, or quitting everything

- Your body is breaking down—more headaches, fatigue, random aches
- You don't feel like "you" anymore

If you felt any of that, it's not just life being hard. You're burnt out. And you deserve to heal. Pause: You Were Never Meant to Live Like This

Let's get something straight:

You were never created to live your entire life in fight, flight, or freeze.

You were not built to:

- Say yes to everything
- Constantly perform for approval
- Ignore your body's signals
- Be accessible 24/7
- Hustle with no breaks
- Survive instead of live

It is not noble to be exhausted.

It is not a badge of honor to neglect yourself. Being burned out isn't a sign you're strong.

It's a sign you've been carrying too much for too long without support.

Why You Haven't Healed Yet Sometimes we don't slow down because:

- We're afraid everything will fall apart without us
- We've tied our worth to being needed
- We feel guilty taking a break when others are struggling
- We were never taught how to rest emotionally, only physically

But this way of living has a cost:

Your peace. Your health. Your joy. And eventually, your identity.

You cannot help anyone, love anyone, or fulfill any purpose if your flame is gone. Self-care isn't about escaping responsibility—it's about preserving longevity.

You Can Recover. Here's How You Start. Burnout doesn't end with a vacation or a night off.

It ends when you stop betraying yourself to keep everything else running.

Here's what healing looks like:

- Telling the truth about where you are
- Admitting you need help or a break without shame
- Creating micro-rest moments during your day
- Saying "not right now" without guilt
- Rebuilding a rhythm of rest that doesn't wait for you to crash

You don't need to disappear to heal—you just need to realign.

And it starts with permitting yourself to stop living like you're a machine.

A Note from Mason

I've been there—functioning, achieving, managing—but feeling hollow. I thought I was being strong.

But what I really was… was surviving. And surviving isn't the same as living.

Burnout taught me something powerful:

If you don't learn to care for yourself, your body and soul will force you to. And when that happens, it's not always gentle.

So don't wait until you break. Start listening now.

Start choosing you now.

Take Care Action Steps

1. Self-Check Inventory: Answer these questions honestly:

- What am I constantly doing that leaves me drained?

- Who or what do I need to say "not right now" to?

- When was the last time I felt truly rested?

2. Body Awareness Moment: Throughout your day, stop and ask:

"What is my body feeling right now? Where am I holding tension?" Then breathe, stretch, or pause—even just for 90 seconds.

3. Write a Burnout Letter:

Write a private letter that starts with: "Dear Burnout..."

Say everything you've been holding in. Be raw. Be real. Burn it if you need to.

4. Create a "No" List:

List 3 things you are no longer available for starting this week.

Example: "I am no longer available for overcommitting, fake friendships, or guilt when I rest."

5. Schedule Recovery Time:

Choose 1 day this month to completely unplug—no work, no pressure, no productivity. Just healing space. Treat it like a meeting with your soul. Don't miss it.

"The most loving word you'll ever learn to say is 'No.'"

Chapter 3

Boundaries Are Not Selfish

You were taught to be nice. To be polite. To be available. To say yes. But nobody ever taught you how to say no with confidence.

No one showed you how to create boundaries without guilt.

And somewhere along the way, you confused people-pleasing with being kind.

But here's the truth:

Boundaries are not selfish, they are survival.

They mark the boundary between safeguarding your peace and sacrificing yourself for others' happiness.

Boundaries are not walls to keep people out. They are doors with locks—to decide who gets access and how often.

What Happens When You Have No Boundaries

When you don't have boundaries, everything in your life feels heavy. You say yes when you want to say no.

You over-explain your decisions to avoid disappointing others. You agree to things you don't have the capacity for.

You tolerate behavior that drains you because you're afraid of conflict. And slowly… you stop recognizing yourself.

Without boundaries:

- You begin to resent the very people you love

- You feel used, overlooked, and invisible

- You become emotionally reactive, not peaceful

- You lose the ability to rest without guilt

- You feel like your life belongs to everyone but you

This is what happens when you confuse being available with being valuable.

Why Setting Boundaries Feels So Hard

Boundaries don't come easy to people who:

- Were raised to be the "responsible one"

- Feel guilty when others are upset

- Grew up in homes where saying no wasn't allowed

- Learned love meant self-sacrifice, even when it hurt

We fear that if we say no:

- They'll leave

- They'll think we're selfish

- We'll look weak or ungrateful

- Conflict will explode

- We'll feel bad for days

But what's worse than feeling guilty for a few minutes? Feeling resentful for a lifetime.

You Are Allowed to Protect Your Energy Let's be clear:

- You are not required to answer every text immediately.

- You are not obligated to attend every event you're invited to.

- You are not wrong for saying, "I need space," "I can't help right now," or "I'm unavailable."

You are allowed to be unavailable.

Your time, energy, and peace are not unlimited resources. They must be managed like anything valuable.

And guess what? Healthy people respect boundaries. People who love you will adjust.

People who benefit from your lack of boundaries will be the ones who complain the most. Let them.

Real Talk: Boundaries Aren't Meant to Keep You Safe from People—They Keep You Safe Within Yourself

Boundaries say:

- "I love you, but I won't betray myself to keep you comfortable."

- "I can support you, but I won't carry what's not mine."

- "I can be kind and still say no."

They are a form of self-respect.

They teach others how to treat you—because you're finally treating yourself with honor.

When you avoid setting boundaries, you silently say to yourself, "Their comfort is more important than my peace."

But no more.

What Boundaries Actually Sound Like

Let's make this practical. Boundaries don't have to be cold or rude. Here are some healthy, respectful ways to reclaim your peace:

- "I'm not available to talk about that right now."

- "I need a day to rest—I'll circle back with you later."

- "I'm not comfortable with that request, and I have to say no."

- "Please don't raise your voice at me. I'm happy to talk when things are calm."

- "That doesn't work for me. Here's what I can offer."

You don't owe long explanations. No is a full sentence.

And when you say it from a place of self-respect—not bitterness—you'll feel power coming back into your hands.

Freedom Through Boundaries

Imagine this:

You wake up without resentment. You go through your day with clarity. You feel peace in your relationships. You feel safe in your own space.

You no longer live in constant emotional reaction mode. That is the freedom boundaries bring.

Boundaries create room for rest. For creativity.

For authenticity.

For real love—not one-sided love based on your constant availability.

A Note from Mason

There were years of my life where I said yes to everything… and no to myself. I was the helper. The fixer. The reliable one.

But behind that smile was fatigue, bitterness, quiet frustration, and worst of all, I was blaming other people for crossing lines I never set in the first place.

It wasn't until I started honoring my own space that I felt the shift. People didn't leave.

The world didn't fall apart.

But my peace? It came back. And it stayed.

So I say this to you with love: You are allowed to protect your energy. You don't have to apologize for taking care of you.

Take Care Action Steps

1. Boundary Inventory:

Write down where in your life you feel the most drained—relationships, work, family, texts, etc. Ask: "What boundary am I afraid to set here?"

2. Your First No:

This week, say no to one thing that you'd normally say yes to out of guilt. Don't overexplain. Just honor your no.

3. Create a Boundary Script:

Choose one phrase that empowers you and practice saying it out loud:

- "Let me get back to you on that."

- "That's not something I can take on right now."

- "I'm not available for that today."

4. Self-Respect Reminder:

Write this down somewhere you'll see it often:

"My peace matters. My time is valuable. I teach others how to treat me by how I treat myself."

5. Protect a Day or Hour Just for You:

This week, block off time where no one gets access to you. No emails. No favors. No obligations. Just space to breathe, rest, or do something that restores you.

"Release the weight that was never yours to carry."

Chapter 4

Letting Go of What's Draining You

Some things in your life were only meant to be temporary.

But you've held on—because you're loyal, hopeful, scared, or unsure of what life would look like without it.

And now?

It's costing you peace. It's stealing your energy. It's blocking your growth. It's weighing you down.

The hard truth?

You cannot heal, rise, or thrive when you're still carrying what's killing your spirit. Letting go is not weakness—it's wisdom. It's strategy. It's self-care.

What's Draining You Isn't Always Obvious

Sometimes what's draining you isn't just toxic people—it's:

- The job you outgrew but won't leave

- The habit you know is slowly ruining your health

- The guilt you keep carrying from a mistake you already apologized for

- The pressure to be perfect

- The constant comparison

- The fake smile you wear every day

Drain doesn't always look dramatic. It looks like:

- Constant brain fog

- Feeling overwhelmed by small tasks

- Being irritable for no reason

- Wanting to disappear for a while

- Losing excitement about the future

- Feeling emotionally flatlined

Your life may not be falling apart.

But something is pulling from you quietly, consistently, relentlessly. And it's time to name it.

Why We Hold On So Long

You know it's draining you, so why do you keep holding on?

- Fear of the unknown – "What if letting go makes things worse?"

- False loyalty – "I've put too much into this to walk away now."

- Guilt – "If I leave, I'll hurt someone."

- Attachment to the memory – "It wasn't always this bad."

- Hope for change – "Maybe it'll get better if I just stick it out."

But ask yourself honestly:

What's the cost of holding on?

If it's draining your joy, your sleep, your sense of self—it's already too expensive.

The Hidden Danger of Emotional Leaks

Think of yourself as a house. Every person, habit, job, or belief is connected to your wiring. If something is faulty—leaking energy—it causes:

- Emotional short-circuiting

- Mental exhaustion

- Spiritual burnout

- Disconnection from your own needs

Some leaks are slow.

A friend who always calls with drama.

A job that praises you but never promotes you. A habit you justify but secretly hate.

The longer you ignore the leak, the more damage it does.

Your emotional power is sacred. Stop letting it drain into broken places. Letting Go is an Act of Self-Respect

Letting go says:

- "I deserve peace more than I deserve to prove a point."

- "I am no longer available for what doesn't love me back."

- "My energy is not free. My future is not negotiable."

You are not a dumpster for guilt, chaos, or unresolved tension. You are a whole person with a future worth protecting.

The strongest thing you can do in some seasons is not fight harder—it's release.

What Letting Go Can Look Like

Letting go doesn't always mean cutting people off or quitting your job overnight. Sometimes it's:

- Releasing expectations that never fit you

- Letting go of roles you played just to be accepted

- Accepting that someone may never apologize

- Freeing yourself from the weight of always being the strong one

- Choosing rest over hustle

- Forgiving yourself for what you didn't know back then

Letting go is emotional surgery.

You're removing what's toxic so the rest of you can breathe again.

A Note From Mason

I didn't know how tired I was until I let go.

I was holding on to people who didn't see me, commitments that didn't align with me, and expectations that didn't fit me. But I called it loyalty. I called it "being strong." I called it "being nice."

But the truth was, I was scared.

Scared to lose, scared to disappoint, scared to start over.

Letting go didn't make me weak. It made me free.

Now I protect my peace like it's gold. Because it is. And you deserve that freedom too.

Take Care Action Steps

1. Energy Audit:

Write down what's draining you. Be honest.

- Who?

- What?

- Where do you feel heaviness after engaging?

2. Release Statement:

Choose one thing from your list and write this:

"I release [insert thing/person/habit] because my peace is more important than my fear."

3. Visual Detox:

Unfollow or mute social media accounts that trigger comparison, anxiety, or emotional fatigue. Your mind deserves better content.

4. Micro-Let-Go Challenge:

Let go of one small thing this week—a plan, an obligation, a grudge. Start small. Feel the shift.

5. Reclaim That Energy:

Use the time or emotional energy you get back to do something that fills you: rest, walk, read, reflect. Replace the drain with delight.

Let's keep going — Chapter 5 is a turning point. We've uncovered the drain... now it's time to reclaim your power. Let's go deep again. 🔥

"Every time you say yes to someone else, make sure you're not saying no to yourself."

Chapter 5

The Power of Saying No

There is a version of you on the other side of "no."

A version that's rested.

A version that's not constantly resentful. A version that feels free—not just busy. A version that finally belongs to you.

But you'll never meet that version if you keep saying yes to everything that steals your time, peace, and purpose.

Saying "no" isn't rejection. It's direction.

It points you back to yourself. Back to clarity. Back to what actually matters.

Why You're Afraid to Say No

Let's be honest: saying no is hard for people who were taught to be peacekeepers, people-pleasers, or providers. You were trained to:

- Make others comfortable

- Avoid conflict at all costs

- Be agreeable, even when it hurts

- Keep the peace, even if you lose yourself

So now?

Saying no feels like you're breaking some invisible rule:

"If I say no, they'll think I don't care." "If I say no, they'll stop needing me." "If I say no, I'll lose the connection."

But here's the truth:

Every time you say "yes" out of guilt, fear, or obligation—you are saying "no" to your own well-being.

What Constant Yeses Cost You

You're not burned out because you're weak.

You're burned out because you keep saying yes when you necessarily need rest.

You say yes to:

- Plans you have no energy for

- People who drain you

- Deadlines you shouldn't have agreed to

- Family members who guilt-trip you

- Being everything to everyone And what do you get in return?

- Exhaustion.

- Bitterness.

- Resentment.

- Distance from your own peace.

Saying "yes" doesn't always make you a good person. Sometimes, it just makes you an exhausted one.

What "No" Really Means Let's reframe it:

- No is not mean. It's mature.

- No doesn't mean you're selfish. It means you're self-aware.

- No is not rejection—it's a redirection to what really matters.

- No is how you protect the "yeses" that actually matter—your purpose, your health, your sanity.

Saying no is how you start choosing you again.

The Hidden Guilt Trap

You might feel guilty the first few times. That's normal. Why? Because you're breaking an internal pattern that says:

- "I'm only valuable when I'm available."

- "If I don't say yes, they won't like me."

- "I'm not allowed to disappoint anyone."

But here's a breakthrough thought:

Guilt doesn't always mean you're doing something wrong. Sometimes it just means you're doing something new.

You're not hurting people by setting limits.

You're just finally acknowledging that your time, energy, and peace are not infinite—and that's okay.

Practice Saying No Without Apology

Here's how to reclaim your no without overexplaining or emotional gymnastics:

- "Thanks for thinking of me, but I won't be able to make it."

- "That's not something I can take on right now."

- "I don't have the capacity for that, but I hope it goes well."

- "No, thank you." (Yes. That's a complete sentence.)

- "I'm choosing to rest instead." No arguing. No guilt. Just clarity.

You're not required to shrink or strain to be accepted.

A Note from Mason

Learning to say no changed my life.

For too long, I thought I had to be everything to everyone. I feared letting people down. I feared looking selfish. But I was dying inside. Quietly.

One day I realized: Nobody is coming to save my peace but me.

So I started saying no—with shaky hands at first. But over time, it felt powerful. Clean. Liberating.

And I discovered something powerful:

The people who love and respect you will adjust.

The ones who don't? Were only there for what they could take from you.

Your "no" is a boundary. A guardrail. A door protecting the home of your soul. Don't let guilt keep you from using it.

Take Care Action Steps

1. Permission Statement: Write this and say it aloud:

"I give myself permission to say no without guilt, fear, or explanation. My no is valid."

2. No List:

Write 3 things you're saying no to this week. Start small if you need to. Example:

- No to staying up late out of habit

- No to conversations that drain me

- No to guilt when I rest

- Practice Your No:

Choose a simple situation (text, invite, request) where you can politely say no. Say it calmly, kindly, and firmly. Watch how much lighter you feel.

3. Energy Audit Follow-Up:

From Chapter 4—look at what's draining you. What are you still saying yes to that needs a no?

4. Affirmation Reminder: Put this somewhere visible:

"I don't have to explain why I need peace. Protecting myself is a full sentence."

"You don't have to collapse to justify rest. It's not a luxury—it's your lifeline."

Chapter 6

Rest Is Productive

Rest is not a reward. It's a requirement.

You don't have to earn it. You don't have to prove you deserve it. You're allowed to rest simply because you're human.

But the world doesn't teach us that, does it? It teaches:

- "Sleep when you're dead."

- "Grind now, shine later."

- "Don't stop. Keep going."

- "You'll lose momentum if you rest."

But let me ask you this:

What good is momentum if it's dragging you toward burnout?

Some of the most exhausted people on this planet are also the most successful—because they never learned how to pause.

Rest is not lazy.

Rest is not weakness. Rest is productive.

The Lie That Keeps You Drained

Somewhere in your journey, someone convinced you that your value is tied to your output. You're productive = You're worthy.

You're helpful = You're needed.

You're busy = You're doing something important. But that's not the truth. That's a trap.

Here's what happens when you live in that lie:

- You feel guilty sitting still.

- You get anxious during downtime.

- You feel behind the moment you unplug.

- You equate exhaustion with excellence.

And the worst part?

Even when you hit your goals, you still don't feel peace—because you never learned or gave yourself permission to pause and enjoy your success.

What Rest Actually Does

Rest isn't just sleep. It's recovery. It's recalibration. It's realignment. True rest:

- Repairs your nervous system

- Improves your focus

- Restores your creativity

- Balances your emotions

- Protects your physical and mental health

- Makes room for joy, not just relief

When you rest, you give your body permission to heal. When you rest, you give your mind space to reset.

When you rest, you remind yourself:

"I don't have to break to be valuable." You Can't Pour from an Empty Cup

We say it all the time, but do we believe it?

You cannot give your best to others when you have nothing left in you. You cannot love fully when your soul is depleted.

You cannot lead clearly when your mind is foggy. You cannot heal while you're still rushing.

Burnout isn't just exhaustion—it's what happens when you ignore or silence the signals for too long. And rest is the resistance that helps you recover.

Rest Is Not Optional — It's Strategic

Here's what successful people won't always tell you:

The real ones? The healthy ones?

The long-lasting ones?

They build rest into their lives on purpose. They disappear before they're drained.

They unplug to stay aligned.

They understand that the reset is what powers the run.

You don't need to crash before you care for yourself.

You don't have to wait for a breakdown to begin protecting your mental health.

Rest before it's urgent. Rest while you still have peace to protect.

What Rest Can Look Like

Not all rest is the same. Here are some ways to rest that go deeper than naps:

- Mental rest: Silence, journaling, unplugging from screens

- Emotional rest: Safe conversations, crying, not being "on"

- Spiritual rest: Stillness, prayer, meditation, nature walks

- Physical rest: Naps, stretching, full sleep cycles

- Creative rest: Consuming art without pressure to produce

- Social rest: Taking a break from people without guilt

Your body knows what you need. But it won't scream until it's desperate. Start listening now.

A Note from Mason

I used to be addicted to the grind.

I wore exhaustion like a trophy. I thought rest meant weakness. That if I slowed down, I'd fall behind. But I didn't realize I was already falling—falling apart internally.

I learned that rest isn't the enemy of progress—it's the foundation of it.

The moment I started honoring my need to rest, everything shifted. My ideas got clearer, my mood got better, my relationships became richer, and most importantly—I finally felt like I could breathe again.

You don't need to prove anything to earn your right to rest.

Your body and soul deserve peace. And you don't have to apologize for that.

Take Care Action Steps

1. Rest Check-In: Ask yourself:

- When was the last time I truly rested—without guilt, without multitasking, without distraction?

- What kind of rest do I need right now—physical, emotional, or mental?

2. Create a Rest Ritual:

Design a weekly non-negotiable rest moment—whether it's Sunday morning, Friday night, or Wednesday afternoon. Put it in your calendar like a business meeting.

3. Unplug Hour:

Choose one hour this week to unplug from screens, work, noise, and other people. Sit with silence. Let your mind breathe.

4. Permission Statement: Write and repeat:

"Rest is not a luxury. Rest is part of my purpose. I give myself permission to slow down without shame."

5. Choose Recovery Over Reward:

This week, don't treat rest as something you earn after being exhausted. Choose to rest before you're empty. Let it be your strategy, not your survival plan.

"You don't need a new life—you need a new lens."

Chapter 7

Rebuilding Your Mindset

Your mind is the control center of your life.

Before anything changes in your habits… Before your peace is protected…

Before your boundaries are respected… Your mindset must be rebuilt.

Because here's the truth:

You can't create a healthy life with a broken thought system. You can't live free while thinking like a prisoner.

You can't rise while repeating lies to yourself.

And the problem?

Most of those lies didn't start with you.

They were planted—by pain, parents, past experiences, pressure, and people who didn't see your worth.

Now, those thoughts have become a loop:

- "I'm not enough."

- "No one cares what I need."

- "If I stop, I'll fall behind."

- "I have to be perfect to be loved."

- "Taking care of myself is selfish."

If you've thought these things... you're not broken. But it's time to rebuild.

The Foundation Is Faulty Every mindset has a blueprint.

And for many of us, that blueprint was built in survival mode.

You were praised for ignoring your needs. Rewarded for pushing through pain.

Taught that strength was silence. Taught that worth was performance.

So now, you feel:

- Guilty when you slow down

- Uncomfortable when you feel peace

- Suspicious of love that doesn't require you to earn it

- Addicted to pressure because pressure is all you've ever known

This is what happens when your mind is wired for survival instead of safety. It protects you—but it also limits you.

You Can't Heal in the Same Mindset That Broke You Let that sink in.

You cannot create a healed, empowered, joyful life if your thoughts are still shaped by trauma, scarcity, shame, or guilt.

You have to renovate your mental space. Tear down what no longer serves you.

Challenge every thought that tells you:

- You don't deserve rest

- You'll never be enough

- You can't afford peace

- You have to carry it all alone

Because if you don't rewire your mind, you'll keep repeating cycles.

What Mindset Rebuilding Looks Like

This isn't just about positive thinking—it's about truthful thinking. It's about catching the lie, interrupting it, and choosing a better truth.

Old Mindset:

"I'm falling behind." Rebuilt Thought:

"I'm aligned with my own timing. Nothing meant for me will miss me."

Old Mindset:

"I have to say yes or I'll disappoint them." Rebuilt Thought:

"My peace matters more than their temporary approval."

Old Mindset:

"If I rest, I'll look lazy." Rebuilt Thought:

"Rest fuels me. When I pause, I come back stronger."

Old Mindset:

"I can't trust people, I always get hurt." Rebuilt Thought:

"Not everyone is safe, but I can learn to set boundaries and build trust slowly."

Rebuilding isn't instant. It's daily.

It's intentional. But it's worth it.

Watch Your Inner Dialogue

Your thoughts shape your reality. If your mind is a garden, your words are the seeds. Ask yourself:

- Do I talk to myself with compassion or criticism?

- Do I rehearse the worst-case scenario or envision a better future?

- Do I replay shame or speak peace?

You are listening to yourself every day.

Make sure the story you're telling is one you actually want to live.

Breaking Mental Strongholds

Some beliefs have lived in your mind so long, they feel like facts. But they're just familiar lies.

- "I have to struggle to succeed."

- "I'm not lovable unless I'm needed."

- "I'm too old to change."

- "This is just how I am."

- "I'll never be enough."

You don't have to entertain those thoughts anymore. You can fire them. Evict them. Replace them.

Start by asking:

Who told me that? And is it actually true?

You'll be surprised how many "truths" crumble under real inspection.

A Note from Mason

There was a time when I was trapped inside my own head.

I smiled on the outside, but mentally, I was drained. Negative thoughts were my soundtrack. I doubted myself daily. I thought healing would come from doing more. Hustling more. Proving more.

But healing didn't come from grinding.

It came from pausing—and challenging my beliefs.

I started catching the lies I was feeding myself.

I started speaking what I wanted to believe, even when it didn't feel true yet. I started showing up differently in my mind… and it changed everything.

Now I know: your life follows the direction of your thoughts.

So if you want peace—rebuild your mindset until peace becomes your default.

Take Care Action Steps

1. Thought Audit:

For one day, write down the repetitive thoughts you notice—especially under stress. Ask: Is this thought helping me or hurting me?

2. Flip the Script:

Choose 3 negative thoughts you often think of. Write them out, then write a truth that replaces each one. Say those truths aloud for the next 7 days.

3. Morning Mindset Check-In: Every morning, ask yourself:

"What kind of person do I want to be today—and what kind of thoughts support that?"

4. Positive Triggers:

Place reminders of truth where you need them—phone wallpaper, sticky notes, journal pages. Write affirmations like:

- "I am worthy of rest."

- "I am not behind."

- "My peace is my priority."

5. Protect Your Mental Diet:

Unfollow accounts, mute conversations, or take breaks from voices that feed fear, shame, or comparison. Your mind deserves better input.

"Your body isn't a problem to fix. It's a miracle to honor."

Chapter 8

Your Body Deserves Love Too

Your body has been with you through everything. Every heartbreak.

Every long night.

Every overextended day. Every stress-filled season. Every fight for your survival.

Every quiet moment when you wanted to give up but didn't.

And yet, many of us treat our bodies like enemies. We criticize them.

We ignore their signals. We push them past limits.

We measure their worth based on appearance instead of appreciation.

But here's the truth:

Your body deserves love, not punishment. Not just when it looks a certain way.

Not just when it performs perfectly.

But always. Because it's yours. Because it's you.

How We Learn to Hate Our Bodies

Most people don't start out hating their bodies. They're taught to.

- Taught to criticize their weight.

- Taught that rest is laziness.

- Taught that beauty = value.

- Taught to ignore pain until it becomes unbearable.

- Taught that their body must be fixed, sculpted, hidden, or starved to be accepted.

- The result?

- You start to disconnect from your own skin.

- You stop listening to the signs of fatigue, tension, and burnout.

- You numb your hunger. You override your exhaustion.

- You try to shrink yourself—physically and emotionally—to fit someone else's idea of "enough." But it's time to take your body back.

Your Body Isn't the Problem

Your body is not a problem to be solved. It's a home to be cared for.

And like any home, if it's mistreated or neglected long enough—it will start to fall apart. But when you tend to it with compassion?

It starts to repair.

To stabilize.

To trust you again.

Because here's the truth most don't say:

You can't fully heal emotionally while treating your body like it's your enemy. Your physical, emotional, mental, and spiritual health are connected.

You are one person, not parts.

Taking care of your body is not vanity—it's vitality.

Listen to What Your Body Is Saying

Your body is always speaking. The question is: are you listening?

- That headache = you need rest.

- That tightness in your chest = you're overwhelmed.

- That shoulder pain = you've been carrying stress too long.

- That brain fog = your body needs stillness.

- That constant fatigue = your boundaries are leaking.

When you start to love your body, you stop treating pain as normal. You stop wearing exhaustion like a badge.

You start honoring your limits—not as weaknesses, but as wisdom.

What Body Love Actually Looks Like

Body love isn't about reaching a perfect number or looking a certain way. It's about learning to live in your body with kindness.

Real body love sounds like:

- "I'm proud of you for getting up today."

- "It's okay to need rest."

- "I hear you. I'm listening."

- "Thank you for carrying me through."

- "I love you—even when I don't feel like it."

It looks like:

- Eating when you're hungry—without shame.

- Moving your body—not to punish it, but to honor it.

- Resting when you're tired—without guilt.

- Wearing clothes that feel good, not just look good.

- Choosing progress over perfection.

Your body doesn't need to be perfect. It just needs to be partnered with.

Reconnecting With Your Body

If you've been disconnected from your body for years—it's okay. You can reconnect slowly.

- Start by breathing deeply and noticing where tension lives.

- Stretch with intention.

- Touch your skin with gentleness.

- Speak to your body like someone you love.

- Treat it like it's worth protecting—because it is.

The way you treat your body reflects what you believe about yourself. And from now on, you choose love.

A Note from Mason

I didn't always treat my body with respect.

I overworked it. Ignored it. Starved it of rest.

I judged it. Compared it. Tried to fix it constantly.

And then… I crashed.

Not just physically, but emotionally.

Because I didn't realize how much I had been neglecting myself—not just mentally, but physically.

Now? I move differently.

Not because I'm trying to be "fit," but because I want to be whole.

I rest, stretch, walk, breathe, and say thank you to a body that's carried me through every hard season.

You deserve that kind of relationship with yourself. Start today.

Take Care Action Steps

1. Mirror Moment:

Stand in front of the mirror. Don't point out flaws. Look yourself in the eye and say:

"Thank you for carrying me. I promise to treat you better."

2. Body Check-In:

Sit quietly for 2 minutes. Ask your body:

Where do I feel tension? What do I need right now?

Then respond with care—rest, movement, stillness, hydration.

3. Move With Kindness:

Choose one form of movement this week not for weight loss, but for joy—walk, stretch, dance, or breathe deeply.

4. Eat to Nourish, Not Punish:

Have one meal this week where you eat slowly, thankfully, and guilt-free. Let it be a love offering, not a transaction.

5. Create a Body Affirmation:

Write an affirmation and place it where you'll see it daily:

"My body is worthy of love, care, and compassion—exactly as it is."

"Peace doesn't shout. You'll find it when you unplug and listen inward."

Chapter 9

Cut the Noise (Digital Detox)

We are more connected than ever — yet somehow more disconnected from ourselves than we've ever been.

Scroll. Click. Swipe. Like. Watch. Repeat.

Every second of every day, your mind is being pulled in a hundred different directions. You wake up to notifications.

You scroll through lives you're not living.

You compare your behind-the-scenes to someone's highlight reel. You spend hours consuming... and wonder why you feel empty.

Let's be real:

The constant noise is numbing your soul.

And if you don't learn how to step away, unplug, and listen inward...

You will keep losing pieces of yourself to screens that were never designed to restore you.

The Digital Overload Is Real

Your brain was never meant to process this much information this fast. Every scroll floods you with:

- Bad news

- Perfect bodies

- Toxic opinions

- Filtered lifestyles

- Fake success

- Unsolicited drama And all of it comes with a cost.

- You might not notice it at first, but it shows up like this:

- You can't focus.

- You feel low but don't know why.

- You compare your life to people you've never met.

- You feel behind, unworthy, uninteresting.

- You avoid silence because silence feels uncomfortable now.

- You numb with content, but never feel truly full.

The truth?

Most of us aren't just addicted to our phones. We're addicted to distraction—because silence would force us to face ourselves.

Constant Input Blocks Inner Clarity

When your brain is filled with everyone else's opinions, desires, highlight reels, and content… You lose touch with your own thoughts.

You stop asking:

- "What do I really want?"

- "What does peace feel like to me?"

- "What does success look like for my life?"

- "What is God, the universe, or my intuition saying to me?" Because noise drowns all of that out.

And here's what you must remember:

Silence is not your enemy. It's your access point to clarity.

What a Digital Detox Actually Means

You don't have to throw your phone in the ocean. This isn't about hating technology.

It's about setting boundaries with the things that control your attention.

It's about becoming aware of:

- What triggers insecurity

- What drains your joy

- What breaks your focus

- What steals your time

- What has more of your mind than your own healing does

You can love being connected and still need breaks. You can be informed and protect your mind.

You can support others without comparing your life to theirs. Signs You Need a Digital Detox

You know it's time when:

- You reach for your phone before your feet hit the floor

- You feel anxious when you're offline for too long

- You've scrolled for hours and still feel empty

- You constantly compare your pace, body, or life to others

- You're consuming more than you're creating

- You feel disconnected from the real world around you

This isn't judgment. This is awareness.

You can't change what you don't acknowledge.

Make Peace Louder Than the Noise

The goal isn't just to reduce screen time.

The goal is to make room for what actually matters:

- Presence

- Stillness

- Real connection

- Inner peace

- Emotional clarity

- Creative flow

- Healing thoughts

You're not meant to live life glued to a feed.

There's more to your life than likes, follows, and views.

And the most real version of you? You meet them in the silence.

A Note from Mason

I had to face it myself:

There were moments I picked up my phone not because I had something to check, but because I was trying to avoid my own thoughts.

I used distraction to escape discomfort.

But the more I escaped, the more I lost sight of what I actually needed.

Eventually, I took a weekend off social media. That turned into a full week. The clarity that came back? Unmatched.

My creativity returned. My anxiety lowered. My energy shifted.

It reminded me of this truth:

Your healing can't go viral. It happens offline. In the quiet. In the real.

You don't have to disappear forever.

But you owe yourself some time without the noise.

Take Care Action Steps

1. Social Scan:

Go through your following list. Mute or unfollow anyone who makes you feel anxious, less than, or distracted from your values.

2. The First Hour Rule:

For the next 3 mornings, don't check your phone for the first hour after you wake up. Instead, pray, breathe, journal, stretch, sit in silence—or just be.

3. The 24-Hour Detox:

Pick one day this week where you go 24 hours with no social media or non-essential apps. Notice how you feel—mentally, emotionally, spiritually.

4. Replace the Scroll:

Keep a book, notebook, or positive playlist close. Every time you instinctively reach for your phone out of habit, do one of these instead.

5. Peace Reminder: Put this somewhere visible:

"Peace doesn't make noise. But it's where my power lives."

"You weren't just born to survive—you were born to live on purpose."

Chapter 10

Reclaiming Joy and Purpose

You weren't just created to survive. You were created to live. Not just to push through pain.

Not just to handle business.

Not just to be responsible, reliable, and strong. But to be joyful.

To be whole. To be free.

To live your life — on purpose, with purpose.

If life has made you numb, distracted, bitter, or just... tired, this is your wake-up call: Joy is not a luxury, purpose is not a fantasy, but both are your birthright.

And now that you've let go of what's draining you?

Now that you've rebuilt your mindset, learned to rest, and started choosing peace? It's time to reclaim what makes you feel alive again.

When Joy Slips Away

You didn't mean to lose your joy. It just... faded.

Somewhere between the deadlines, the heartbreak, the responsibilities, and the unspoken pain—you got disconnected from you.

Joy got buried under stress.

Purpose got drowned out by pressure. Fun felt selfish.

Dreams felt childish.

You became who you needed to be to survive—but lost sight of who you were created to be. Let's bring them back.

What Joy Really Is Joy isn't hype.

It's not fake positivity.

It's not surface-level smiles.

Joy is a deep, unshakable sense of aliveness, even when everything isn't perfect.

Joy says:

- "I can breathe again."

- "I feel like myself."

- "I'm not just functioning — I'm living."

- "This feels right, even if it's simple." And here's the key:

You don't wait for joy. You create it. You choose it. You protect it.

Rediscovering Purpose Isn't a One-Time Moment — It's a Daily Choice Purpose isn't some magical job title or viral brand.

It's not just a dream or assignment. Purpose is the reason behind what you do.

You could be:

- A teacher changing the way kids see themselves

- A father raising emotionally healthy boys

- An artist creating beauty that heals people

- A coach, a friend, a creator, a business owner, a peacemaker… It's not always loud. But it's always powerful.

You feel purpose when you're doing something that makes your soul say: This is why I'm here.

And the beautiful part?

You don't have to search for purpose outside of yourself.

It's already in you — underneath the pain, underneath the noise, waiting for permission to breathe again.

Joy + Purpose = Fuel for the New You

When you combine joy and purpose, you stop settling. You stop just "getting through life."

You start waking up with intention.

That doesn't mean everything's perfect. It means you're finally aligned.

Aligned with peace. Aligned with your values.

Aligned with what sets your soul on fire.

You take care of yourself best when you're living from a place of joy and purpose—not just survival.

How to Reclaim Joy and Purpose (For Real)

This isn't about dramatic life overhauls. It's about reconnecting with what matters most — little by little, moment by moment.

Ask yourself:

- What makes me feel light again?

- What did I stop doing that I used to love?

- What brings me peace — not pressure?

- Who am I when I'm not trying to impress or perform?

- What do I want my life to say when it's all said and done?

Start there. Follow the spark.

Joy and purpose will meet you along the way.

A Note from Mason

There was a time when I thought joy was something I'd get to after the hard part was over. That purpose was something for other people who had it all together.

But here's what I've learned:

Joy is part of the healing. And purpose doesn't wait for perfection.

I found both when I slowed down. When I listened inward.

When I stopped performing and started living.

Now I guard them with everything in me. And I want you to do the same.

You've been through enough. Now it's time to live.

With joy. With clarity. With fire in your belly and peace in your soul.

You matter.

Your story matters.

And your next chapter is still being written.

Write it well. On purpose.

Take Care Action Steps

1. Joy Journal:

Make a list of 10 things that make you feel joy — big or small. Commit to doing at least one this
week just because it makes you feel alive.

2. Purpose Check-In:

Write a one-sentence answer to this question:

"What do I feel called to do in this season, even if it's small?"

3. Reclaim a Forgotten Dream:

Revisit something you used to love or dream about that life pushed aside. Take one step toward it

— even if it's just writing it down again.

4. Define Your New Normal: Journal this:

"What does a joyful, purposeful life look like for me — and what's one small change I can make
to move toward it?"

5. Final Declaration: Write it, say it, believe it:

"I am done surviving. I am choosing to live with joy, peace, and purpose. Starting now."

Thank you for reading Take Care of Yourself. This is more than a book it's your comeback. I want
to leave you with a 30-day challenge. Enjoy my friend until we connect again.

30 Days To Take Care Of Yourself

A Self-Care Challenge to Heal, Reset, and Reclaim Your Peace Day 1: Breathe

Take 5 deep breaths and sit in silence for 2 minutes.

Day 2: Digital Detox

Log off social media for 3 hours.

Day 3: Gratitude

Write down 3 things you' are thankful for.

Day 4: Boundaries

Say no to one thing that drains you today.

Day 5: Hydration

Drink at least 64 oz of water.

Day 6: Rest

Take a 20-minute nap or lie down without distraction.

Day 7: Movement

Stretch for 10 minutes or take a walk.

Day 8: Unplug

No screens 30 minutes before bed.

Day 9: Encouragement

Text or call someone and encourage them. Day 10: Declutter

Tidy up one small space (desk, drawer, or room).

Day 11: Mindfulness

Notice your thoughts without judgment.

Day 12: Nature

Spend 15 minutes outside.

Day 13: Journaling

Write what's been weighing on your mind.

Day 14: Affirmations

Say 5 positive things about yourself.

Day 15: Silence

Take 10 minutes in complete silence.

Day 16: Disconnect

Turn your phone off for 1 hour.

Day 17: Self-talk

Catch and correct one negative thought.

Day 18: Laugh

Watch or read something that makes you laugh.

Day 19: Nourish

Eat something that makes your body feel good.

Day 20: Revisit a Hobby

Do something creative or fun.

Day 21: Breathe Again

Try 4-4-4-4 breathing (box breathing).

Day 22: Reflect

Write one thing you've learned about yourself.

Day 23: Encourage Yourself Write a letter to your future self.

Day 24: Music

Listen to music that uplifts you.

Day 25: Forgive

Release one person in your heart today.

Day 26: Speak Life

Speak three declarations over yourself.

Day 27: Joy

Do something fun just because.

Day 28: Plan

Schedule rest into your upcoming week.

Day 29: Stretch

Move gently and thank your body.

Day 30: Celebrate

Celebrate your growth and commit to continuing.

Bonus Workbook: Your Personal Self-Care Reset

1. The "No Guilt" Self-Care Checklist

☑ Took 5 Took 5 deep breaths intentionally

☑ Said "no" to something I didn't have the capacity for

☑ Drank water before caffeine

☑ Gave myself permission to rest

☑ Spent time offline without FOMO

☑ Affirmed myself out loud

☑ Released someone or something mentally

☑ Took a walk or stretched

☑ Smiled or laughed for no reason

☑ Celebrated a small win

How many did you check off? Circle one: ☐ 1-3 ☐ 4-6 ☐ 7-10

➡ Write one feeling you're leaving behind: _____

➡ Write one word you're taking into your next week: _____

2. **Weekly Self-Care Planner**

Day   **One Thing I'll Do to Take Care of Me**

Monday

Tuesday

Wednesday

Thursday

Friday

Saturday

Sunday

3. **Journal Prompt: My Peace Plan**

"When I feel overwhelmed, I will..."

_____

"I know I'm at peace when..."

_____

"I commit to protecting my peace by..."

_____

4. Build Your Own Affirmations

I am worthy of _____

I am learning to _____

I am releasing _____

I am showing up for myself by _____

I choose peace over _____

5. 7-Day Self-Care Reset

Day	Focus	What I Did or Noticed
1	Rest	
2	Boundaries	
3	Mindset Shift	
4	Body Awareness	
5	Digital Detox	
6	Joy Activity	
7	Gratitude + Peace	

You don't need to have it all figured out. Just start where you are and take care of you—one breath, one boundary, one "no," one "yes," at a time.

Acknowledgments

To everyone who has ever felt invisible, exhausted, or empty from constantly showing up for others — this book was written for you. Thank you for your quiet strength, your hidden tears, and your resilience.

To the team at Eagle Eye Press, thank you for believing in the power of real stories and honest healing.

And to the reader — thank you for trusting me with your time and your healing. My hope is that these pages gave you what the world often forgets to give: permission to pause, breathe, and take care of yourself.

About The Author

Mason Reed is a writer, thinker, and voice for those quietly fighting burnout and overwhelmed behind the scenes. Known for his honest, compassionate, and no-fluff approach, Mason speaks to the soul of readers who need to slow down, break cycles, and finally choose themselves.

When he's not writing, he's resting, healing, walking in nature, and protecting his peace like his life depends on it—because it does. He resides in Florida with his wife, Linda, and their three children: Max, Bobby, and Patty.

Connect With Mason Reed

Let's stay connected. Follow Mason for daily encouragement, book updates, and upcoming releases:

Instagram: @masonreedbooks

X @masonreedbooks